I0410686

Ketogenic Diet

Quick and Easy Ketogenic Diet Recipes For Fast Weight Loss

Stella Parker

Table of Contents

INTRODUCTION

Thank you for purchasing this book. It is my pleasure to introduce you to the Ketogenic Meat Cookbook and help you to make many new delicious recipes.

❖ What is the ketogenic diet?

The ketogenic diet is low carb, high fat, and adequate protein diet. This diet helps to burn fat instead of carbohydrates for energy. The body converts carbohydrates into glucose which is then used as energy throughout the body. The ketogenic diet does lower your carb intake so that your body can go into survival mode and convert stored fat into energy. This state is called ketosis. During ketosis, your body produce ketones, which are created from the fats that are broken down in the liver. The primary aim of the ketogenic diet is to make your body go into this metabolic state in order to gain certain health benefits as well as to shape your body. By following the ketogenic diet, you will be able to achieve successful weight loss due to the metabolic advantage of a low carb diet. The ketogenic diet is not only for weight loss. In fact, it has other benefits like it helps relieve acid reflux, helps to slow down certain nerve related diseases, and also helps to slow the physical results of aging. This book contains delicious recipes. Each recipe has nutrition info, which tells you what you are eating every meal and helps you control your weight.

Thank you so much for reading this book!
I hope this book is able to teach you how the ketogenic diet can simplify your everyday life.

Chapter one Fish Recipes

1-Crunchy Crusted Salmon

Total Time: 20 minutes

Serves: 4 Servings

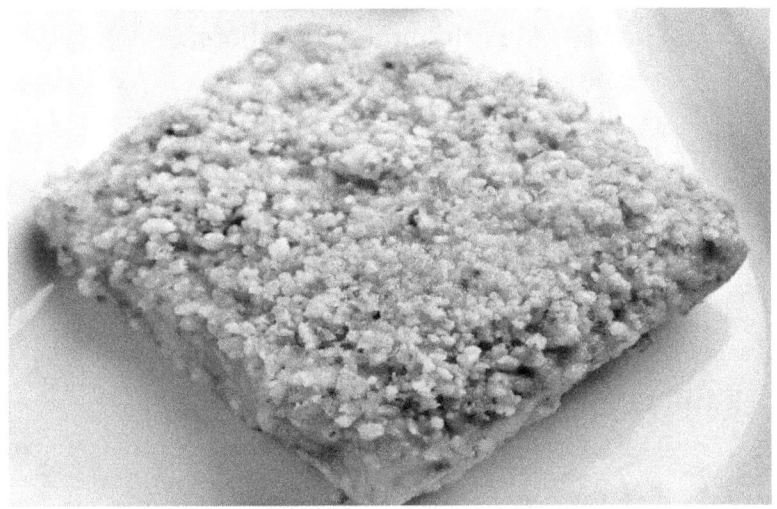

Ingredients:
- 4 salmon fillets
- 2 tablespoon olive oil
- Pepper and salt, for taste
- For crunchy crust:
- 1 tsp coconut amino
- 1 tablespoon vinegar
- 2 1/2 tablespoon maple syrup
- 1/2 tsp onion powder

- 1/2 cup walnuts, chopped
- 1 tsp paprika
- 1/2 chipotle powder
- 1/2 pepper

Directions:
1. In a small bowl, add all crust ingredients and mix well until combined.
2. Place the salmon fillets in a dish and spoon the crust mixture evenly onto each fillet.
3. Place in the refrigerator for 2 hours.
4. Preheat the oven to 425 F.
5. Heat olive oil in a large pan over high heat.
6. Once the pan is hot, then add the fish fillets and cook for 2 minutes.
7. Place pan in preheated oven and cook for 6 minutes.
8. Serve warm and enjoy.

Nutritional Value (Amount per Serving):
- Calories 428
- Fat 27.3 g
- Carbohydrates 10.5 g
- Sugar 7.8 g
- Protein 38.4 g
- Cholesterol 78 mg

2-Quick and Easy Lime Salmon

Total Time: 15 minutes

Serves: 3 Servings

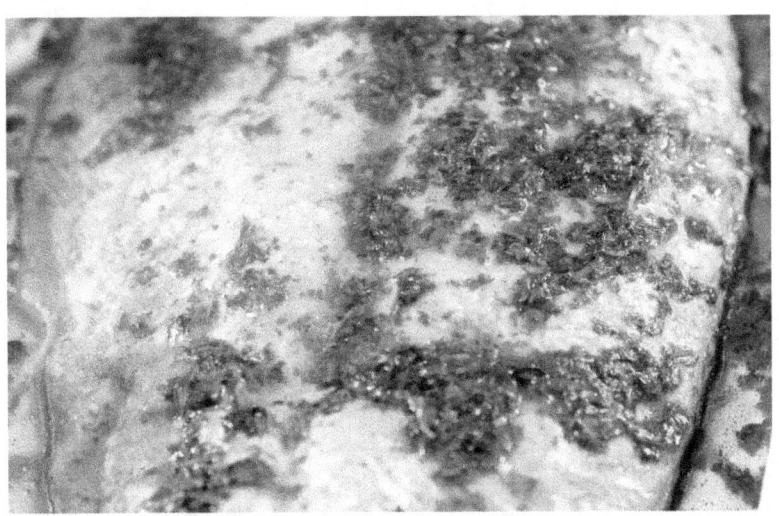

Ingredients:
- 1 lb salmon fillet
- 1 garlic clove, chopped
- 1 tablespoon cilantro, chopped
- Juice and zest of 1/2 lime
- 1 tablespoon olive oil
- Pepper
- Salt

Directions:
1. Preheat the oven to 400 F.

2. Add garlic, cilantro, lemon zest, lemon juice and oil in blender and blend until smooth.
3. Place salmon on baking tray and season with pepper and salt.
4. Spread lime mixture on salmon fillet evenly and bake in preheated oven for 10 minutes.
5. Serve and enjoy.

Nutritional Value (Amount per Serving):
- Calories 242
- Fat 14.0 g
- Carbohydrates 0.4 g
- Sugar 0.2 g
- Protein 29.4 g
- Cholesterol 67 mg

3-Delicious Baked Cod

Total Time: 30 minutes

Serves: 4 Servings

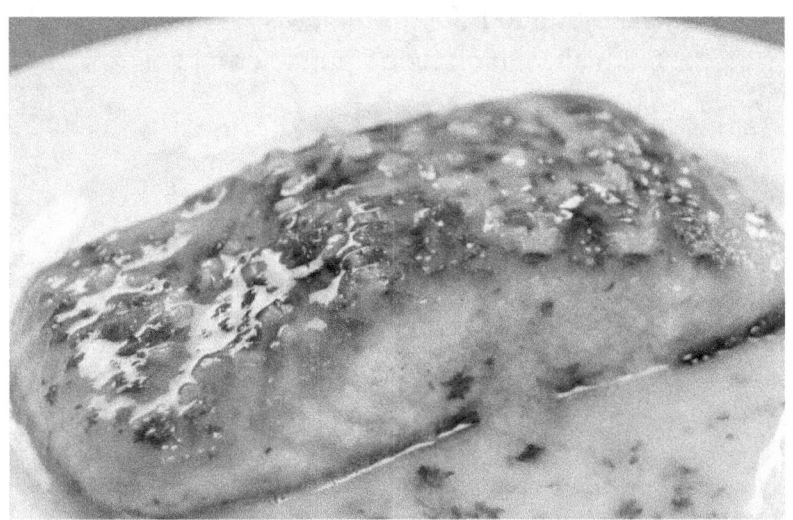

Ingredients:
- 2 lbs cod fillet
- 1/4 tsp paprika
- 4 tablespoon all purpose flour
- 2 tablespoon fresh lemon juice
- 4 tablespoon butter, melted
- Freshly chopped parsley, for garnish
- Pepper
- Salt

Directions:
1. Combine lemon juice and melted butter.

2. In a shallow dish Combine flour, pepper and salt.
3. First dip fish into lemon butter mixture then coat with flour mixture.
4. Place coated fish on baking tray. Sprinkle paprika over fish fillets.
5. Bake at 350 F for 25 minutes.
6. Garnish with chopped parsley and serve.

Nutritional Value (Amount per Serving):
- Calories 371
- Fat 13.6 g
- Carbohydrates 6.2 g
- Sugar 0.1 g
- Protein 52.8 g
- Cholesterol 155 mg

4-Creamy Fish Chowder

Total Time: 30 minutes

Serves: 5 Servings

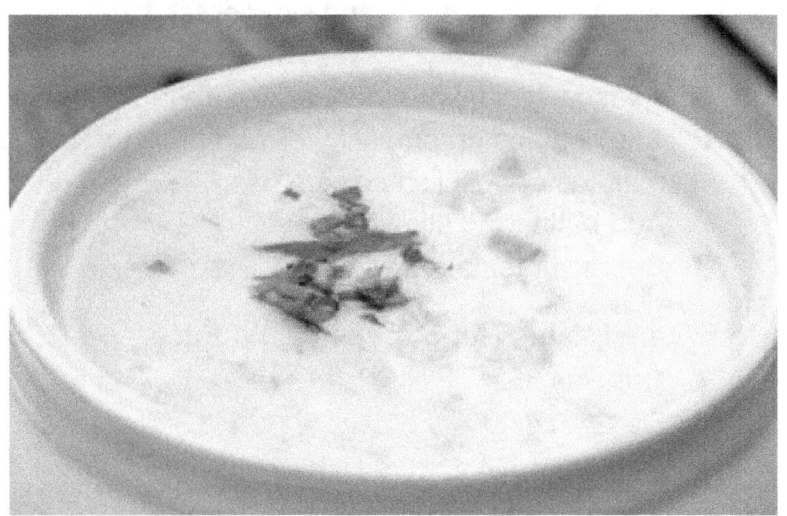

Ingredients:
- 1 lb white fish, chopped
- 1 tablespoon butter
- 2 cups heavy cream
- 1/2 tsp thyme, dried
- 2 1/2 cups vegetable stock
- 3 cups daikon radish, chopped
- 1 medium onion, chopped
- 3 bacon slices, chopped
- Pepper
- Salt

Directions:

1. Cook bacon in a pan over medium heat until crisp.
2. Remove bacon from pan and place on a plate.
3. Add daikon radish and onion to bacon grease pan and cook for 10 minutes.
4. Add vegetable stock and simmer for 10 minutes.
5. Season with thyme, pepper and salt.
6. Add fish and cream, stir well and cook for 4 minutes or until fish cooked.
7. Add butter and stir well.
8. Serve immediately and enjoy.

Nutritional Value (Amount per Serving):

- Calories 362
- Fat 27.0 g
- Carbohydrates 5.8 g
- Sugar 2.3 g
- Protein 23.9 g
- Cholesterol 142 mg

5-Simple Grilled Tilapia

Total Time: 15 minutes

Serves: 6 Servings

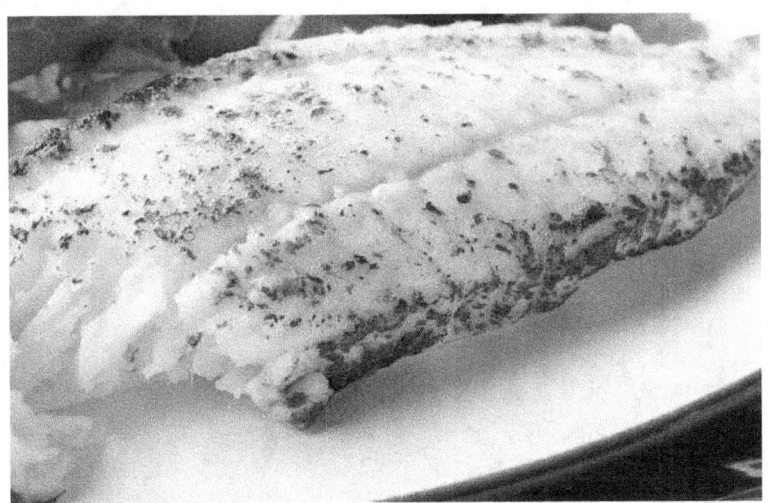

Ingredients:
- 2 lbs tilapia fillets
- 1 tsp garlic powder
- 1/2 fresh lemon juice
- 1 tablespoon butter, melted
- Pepper
- Salt

Directions:
1. Preheat the grill on high.

2. In a small bowl, combine lemon juice, garlic powder and butter and microwave for 10 seconds.
3. Brush both sides of the fish fillet with the lemon mixture.
4. Season fillet with pepper and salt to taste.
5. Spray grill with cooking spray.
6. Place fillets on preheated grill and grill for 4 minutes on each side.
7. Serve hot and enjoy.

Nutritional Value (Amount per Serving):
- Calories 143
- Fat 3.3 g
- Carbohydrates 0.4 g
- Sugar 0.1 g
- Protein 28.2 g
- Cholesterol 79 mg

6-Yummy Pineapple Tuna Burgers

Total Time: 45 minutes

Serves: 4 Servings

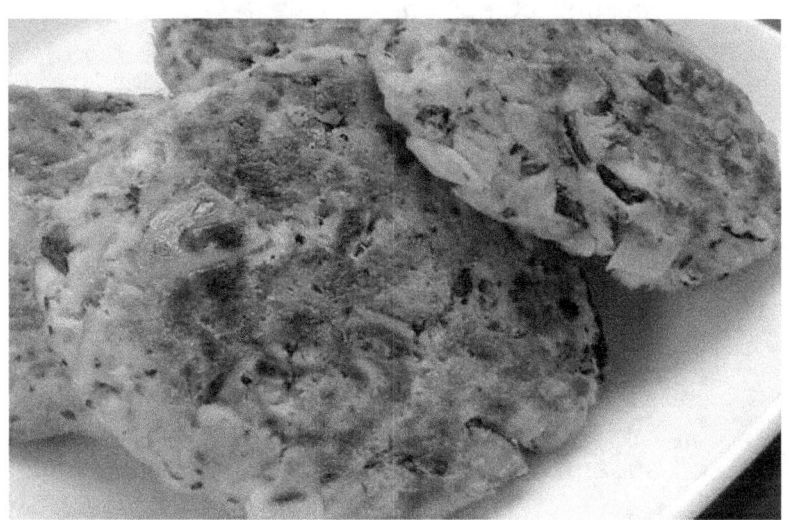

Ingredients:
- 2 cans tuna
- 1/2 tablespoon fresh lime juice
- 1 large egg
- 4 tablespoon almond flour
- 1/2 cup cilantro, chopped
- 1 can pineapple, crushed and drained
- 1/4 tsp chili flakes
- 1/4 tsp ground ginger
- 2 garlic cloves
- 1 tablespoon soy sauce

- Pepper
- Salt

Directions:
1. Preheat the oven to 400 F.
2. In a mixing bowl, add all ingredients and mix well until combined.
3. Make four equal patties from mixture.
4. Place patties on baking dish and bake in preheated oven for 25 minutes.
5. Turn patties and bake for another 10 minutes.
6. Serve and enjoy.

Nutritional Value (Amount per Serving):
- Calories 189
- Fat 8.5 g
- Carbohydrates 1.1 g
- Sugar 0.1 g
- Protein 25.6 g
- Cholesterol 74 mg

7-Tasty Cheese Crusted Tilapia

Total Time: 20 minutes

Serves: 4 Servings

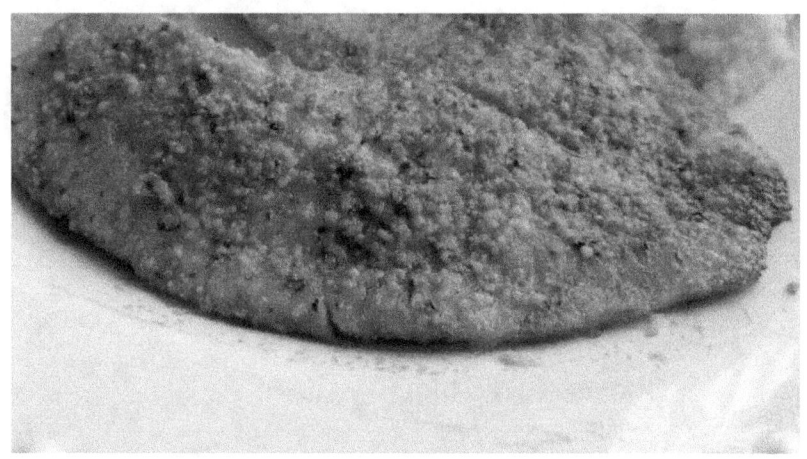

Ingredients:
- 4 tilapia fillets
- 1 tablespoon olive oil
- 1 tablespoon fresh parsley, chopped
- 2 tsp paprika
- 3/4 cup parmesan cheese, grated
- 1/4 tsp salt

Directions:
1. Preheat the oven at 400 F.
2. Spray baking dish with cooking spray and set aside.

3. In a bowl, combine parsley, cheese, paprika and salt.
4. Drizzle fish fillet with olive oil then dip into cheese mixture and place on prepared baking dish.
5. Place in preheated oven and bake for 10 minutes.
6. Serve and enjoy.

Nutritional Value (Amount per Serving):
- Calories 127
- Fat 4.7 g
- Carbohydrates 0.6 g
- Sugar 0.2 g
- Protein 21.3 g
- Cholesterol 55 mg

Chapter two Pork Recipes

8-Low Carb Pork Chops

Total Time: 35 minutes

Serves: 6 Servings

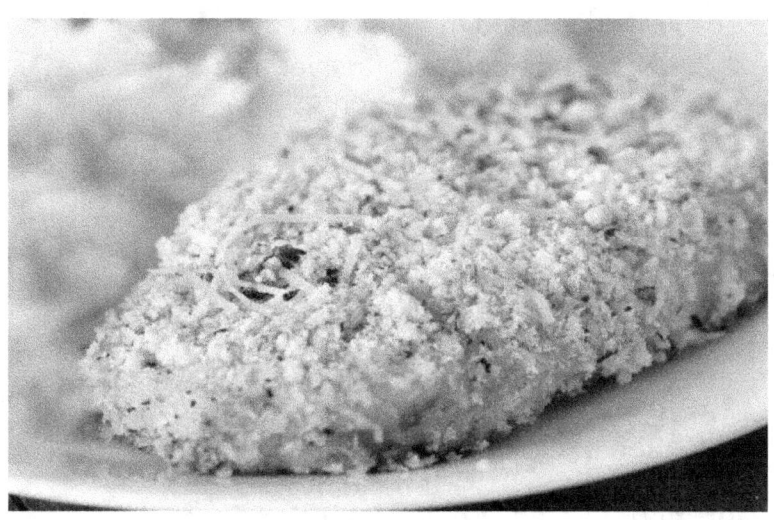

Ingredients:
- 6 thin pork chops, boneless
- 1 1/2 cups parmesan cheese, grated
- 1/2 tsp basil, dried
- 1/2 tsp oregano, dried
- 1/2 tsp onion powder
- 1/2 tsp thyme
- 1/2 tsp garlic powder
- 1/2 tsp pepper

- 5 tablespoon Dijon mustard
- 3 tablespoon extra virgin olive oil
- 1/2 tsp salt

Directions:

1. In a small bowl, combine basil, oregano, onion powder, thyme, garlic powder, olive oil, mustard, 1/4 tsp pepper and 1/4 tsp salt.
2. Add pork chops in large mixing bowl. Pour marinade and mix well until combined.
3. Place in refrigerator for overnight.
4. Preheat the oven to 400 F.
5. Place parmesan cheese in shallow dish.
6. Coat each pork chop with cheese make sure all sides are well coated.
7. Place coated pork chops in a roasting pan.
8. Season pork chops with remaining pepper and salt.
9. Bake in preheated oven for 20 minutes.
10. Serve and enjoy.

Nutritional Value (Amount per Serving):

- Calories 327
- Fat 27.4 g
- Carbohydrates 1.3 g
- Sugar 0 g
- Protein 18.7 g
- Cholesterol 69 mg

9-Delicious Pork Stir Fry

Total Time: 25 minutes

Serves: 4 Servings

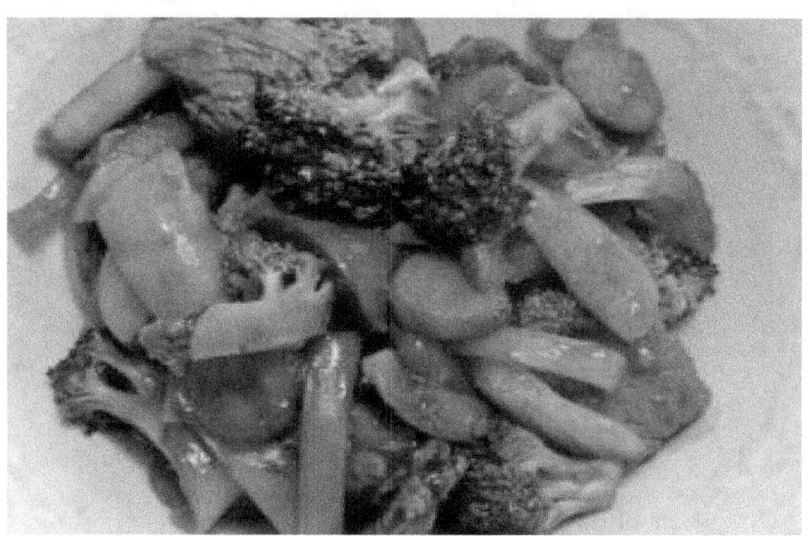

Ingredients:
- 1 lb pork, cut into pieces
- 1 tablespoon cornstarch
- 1 cup chicken broth
- 1/2 tsp ground ginger
- 1/8 tsp red chili flakes
- 1 tablespoon extra virgin olive oil
- 3 tablespoon soy sauce
- 1 medium onion, sliced
- 16 oz frozen broccoli

Directions:

1. Spray pan with cooking spray.
2. Add onion and broccoli and cook over medium-high heat for minutes or until onion soften. Remove from pan and set aside.
3. In a small bowl, combine cornstarch, chicken broth, soy sauce and red chili flakes.
4. Add olive oil in a pan and reduce heat to medium.
5. Add ground ginger and pork. Mix well and cook about 4 minutes, turn pork pieces and cook another minute.
6. Pour cornstarch mixture and stir well.
7. Add cooked onion and broccoli, stir well and cook for minutes.
8. Serve hot and enjoy.

Nutritional Value (Amount per Serving):
- Calories 266
- Fat 8.2 g
- Carbohydrates 13.2 g
- Sugar 3.5 g
- Protein 35.2 g
- Cholesterol 83 mg

10-asty Dijon Herb Pork Tenderloin

Total Time: 30 minutes

Serves: 6 Servings

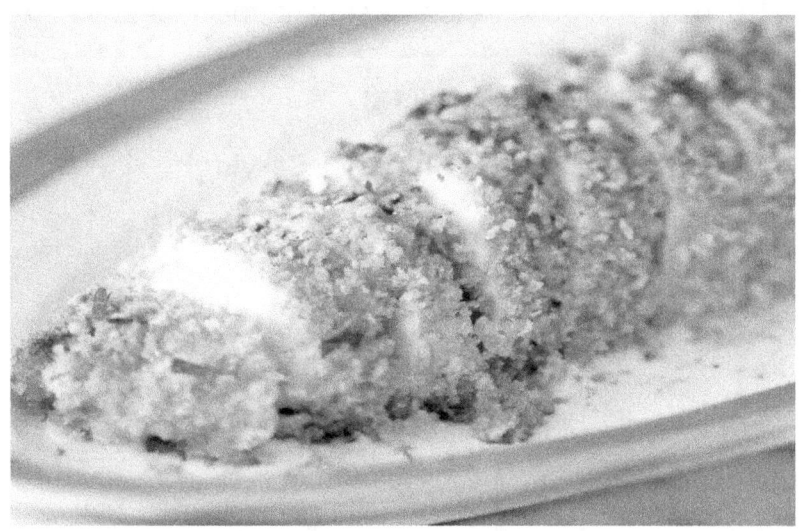

Ingredients:
- 1 lb pork tenderloin
- 2 tablespoon Dijon mustard
- 1/2 tsp rosemary, dried
- 1/2 tsp thyme, dried
- 1 tablespoon olive oil
- 2 tablespoon garlic, minced
- 1/4 tsp pepper
- 1/4 tsp salt

Directions:
1. Preheat the oven to 425 F.

2. Spray a baking tray with cooking spray and set aside.
3. In a small bowl, combine rosemary, thyme, olive oil, garlic, pepper, and salt.
4. Brush tenderloin with mustard then rub with herb mixture.
5. Place in preheated oven and roast for 25 to 30 minutes.
6. Cut into slices and serve.

Nutritional Value (Amount per Serving):
- Calories 273
- Fat 10.5 g
- Carbohydrates 2.8 g
- Sugar 0.2 g
- Protein 40.4 g
- Cholesterol 110 mg

11-Low Carb Grilled Pork

Total Time: 35 minutes

Serves: 4 Servings

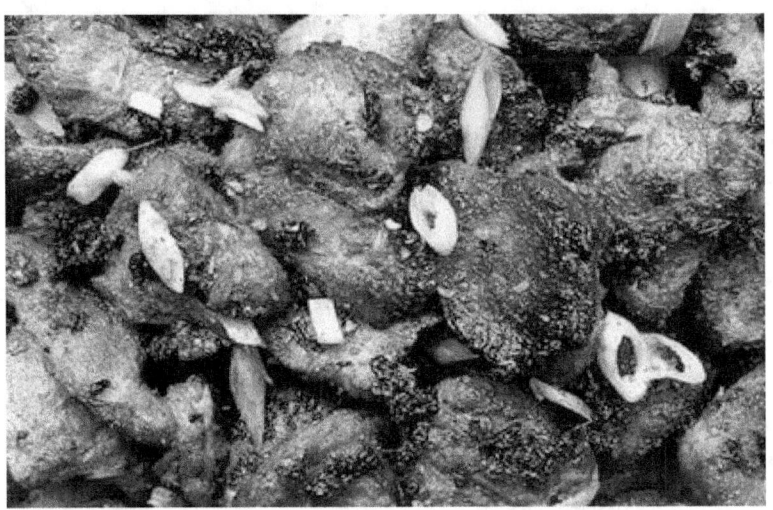

Ingredients:
- 2 lbs pork shoulder, sliced
- 1 fresh lime juice
- 1 tsp water
- 3 tsp honey
- 3 tablespoon olive oil
- 4 tablespoon fish sauce
- 2 tablespoon coconut amino
- 2 stalks lemongrass, cut top and bottom
- 1 large shallot
- 5 garlic cloves

Directions:
1. Add lemongrass, olive oil, fish sauce, coconut amino, shallot and cloves in food processor and process until fine mixture.
2. Pour lemongrass mixture over sliced pork. Mix well and refrigerate overnight.
3. Remove marinated pork from the refrigerator 1 hour before cooking.
4. Preheat grill over medium-high heat.
5. Place marinated pork slices over preheated grill and grill for 3 minutes per side.
6. Combine honey and water.
7. Brush honey and water mixture over pork slices and grill pork slices another 2 minutes or until golden brown.
8. Serve hot with lime juice and enjoy.

Nutritional Value (Amount per Serving):
- Calories 780
- Fat 59.0 g
- Carbohydrates 6.2 g
- Sugar 5.0 g
- Protein 54.0 g
- Cholesterol 204 mg

12-Creamy Pork Cutlet

Total Time: 20 minutes

Serves: 4 Servings

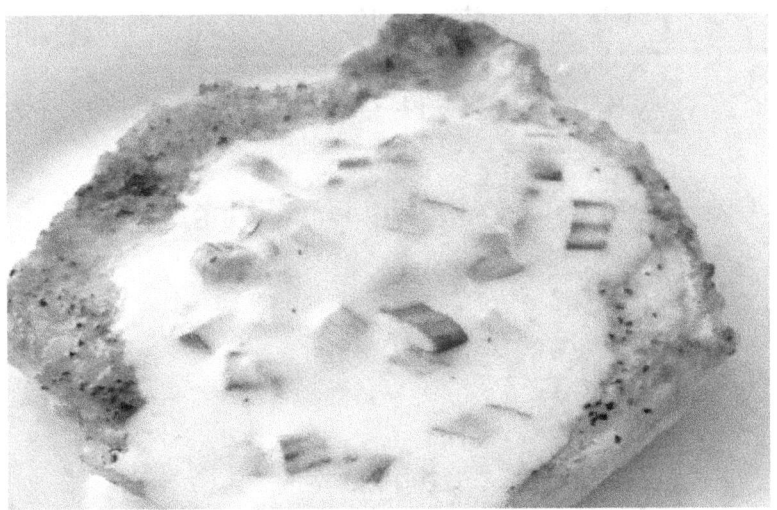

Ingredients:
- 1 1/2 lbs pork, sliced thinly
- 1 fresh lemon juice
- 1/2 cup heavy whipping cream
- 2 green onion, chopped
- 2 tablespoon butter
- Pepper
- Salt

Directions:
1. Season pork slices with pepper and salt.

2. In a small pan, melt 1 tablespoon butter over medium heat once butter melted add onion and sauté for 4 minutes.
3. Add whipping cream stir well and simmer for 10 minutes.
4. In another pan add butter over medium-high heat once butter melted add pork slices and cook for 2 minutes on each side.
5. Add fresh lemon juice to sauce and stir well.
6. Pour sauce over pork slices and serve.

Nutritional Value (Amount per Serving):
- Calories 348
- Fat 17.3 g
- Carbohydrates 1.0 g
- Sugar 0.2 g
- Protein 45.0 g
- Cholesterol 160 mg

13-Delicious Low Carb Pork Soup

Total Time: 4 hours 30 minutes

Serves: 4 Servings

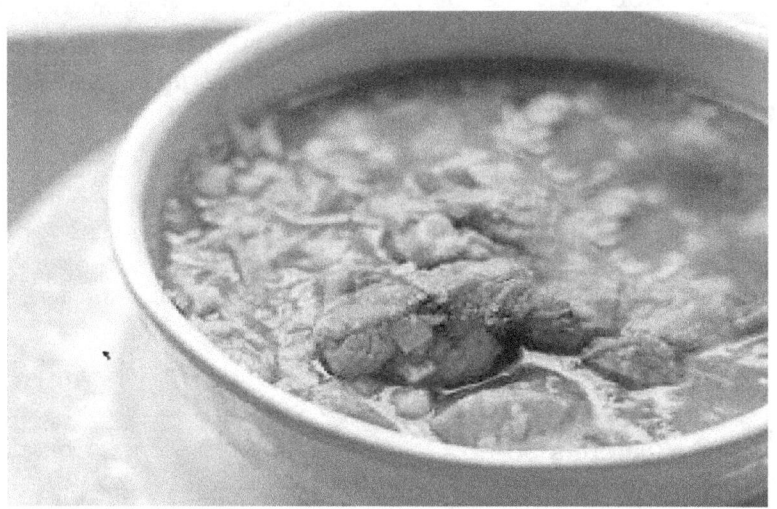

Ingredients:
- 1 lb pork ribs, boneless and cut into 1 inch pieces
- 1 cup cauliflower rice
- 1 tablespoon oregano, chopped
- 1/2 cup water
- 1 cup tomatoes, chopped
- 1/2 cup vegetable stock
- 4 tablespoon dry white wine
- 4 tablespoon onion, chopped
- 1/2 tablespoon garlic, chopped
- 1/2 tablespoon olive oil

- Pepper
- Salt

Directions:
1. Heat olive oil in saucepan over medium heat.
2. Season pork with pepper and salt.
3. Add pork in saucepan and cook until meat becomes brown.
4. Add tomatoes, vegetable stock, white wine and water. Bring to boil.
5. Pour pork mixture into the slow cooker and cook on high for 4 hours.
6. In the last 15 minutes of cooking add cauliflower rice and oregano, stir well.
7. Serve hot and enjoy.

Nutritional Value (Amount per Serving):
- Calories 354
- Fat 22.1 g
- Carbohydrates 4.2 g
- Sugar 1.8 g
- Protein 30.8 g
- Cholesterol 117 mg

14-Slow Cooker Shredded Pork

Total Time: 4 hours 10 minutes

Serves: 5 Servings

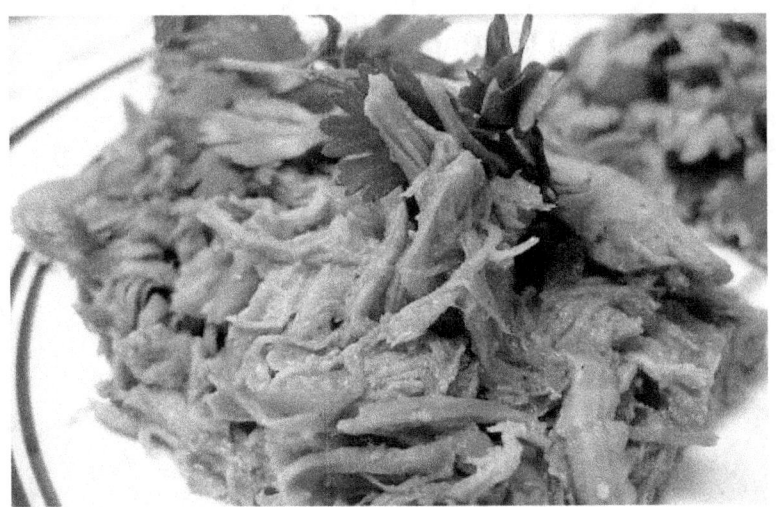

Ingredients:
- 2 lbs pork sirloin roast
- 6 tablespoon cilantro, chopped
- 3/4 tablespoon cumin
- 1 tablespoon chili powder
- 3 tablespoon fresh lime juice
- 1 1/2 tsp kosher salt

Directions:
1. Add all ingredients except cilantro into the slow cooker and mix well.

2. Seal slow cooker with lid and cook on high for 4 hours.
3. Remove pork from slow cooker and shred using a fork.
4. Add cilantro and mix well.
5. Serve with salad and enjoy.

Nutritional Value (Amount per Serving):

- Calories 384
- Fat 17.6 g
- Carbohydrates 1.3 g
- Sugar 0.1 g
- Protein 52.1 g
- Cholesterol 156 mg

Chapter three Chicken Recipes

15-Yummy Baked Chicken

Total Time: 45 minutes

Serves: 4 Servings

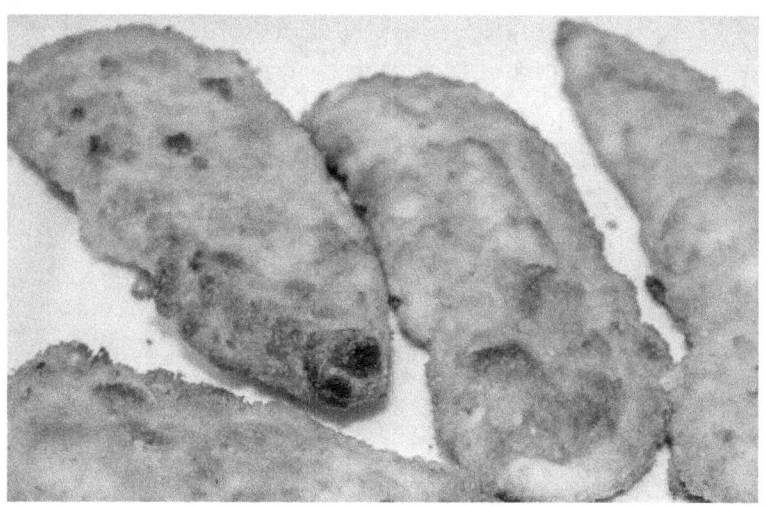

Ingredients:
- 4 chicken breast, skinless and boneless
- 1/2 tsp garlic powder
- 4 tsp breadcrumbs
- 1/2 cup parmesan cheese, shredded
- 1/2 cup mayonnaise
- 1/2 tsp pepper
- 1/4 tsp salt

Directions:

1. Preheat the oven to 400 F.
2. In a small bowl, combine cheese, garlic powder, and mayonnaise.
3. Spray baking tray with cooking spray.
4. Place chicken breast on a baking tray and spread mayonnaise mixture over chicken evenly.
5. Season with pepper and salt.
6. Bake in preheated oven for 20 minutes.
7. After 20 minutes remove chicken from oven and sprinkle breadcrumbs over the top of chicken.
8. Return chicken to the oven and bake for another 20 minutes.
9. Serve hot and enjoy.

Nutritional Value (Amount per Serving):
- Calories 292
- Fat 16.5 g
- Carbohydrates 9.1 g
- Sugar 2.1 g
- Protein 25.7 g
- Cholesterol 83 mg

16-Easy Low Carb Chicken Meatballs

Total Time: 20 minutes

Serves: 3 Servings

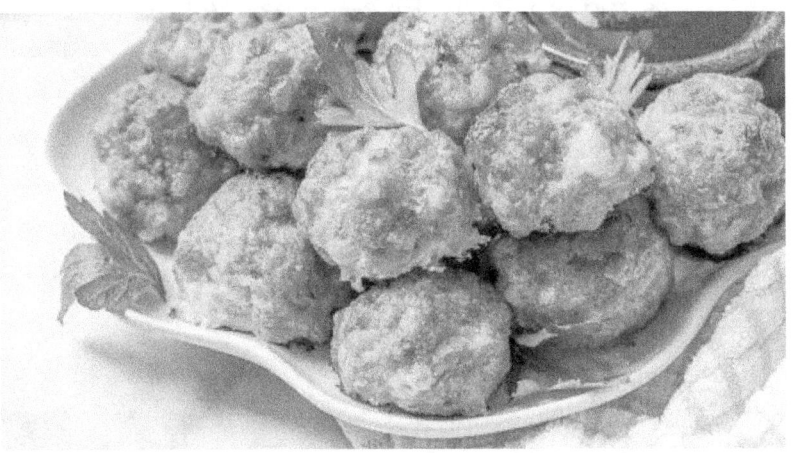

Ingredients:
- 1 lb ground chicken
- 1 large egg
- 4 tablespoon hot sauce
- 4 tablespoon ranch dressing
- 4 tsp cheddar cheese, grated
- 1/2 cup almond flour
- 1/4 cup hot sauce for serving
- Freshly chopped parsley

Directions:
1. Preheat the oven to 500 F.

2. Spray a baking tray with cooking spray and set aside.
3. In mixing bowl, combine chicken, almond flour, cheddar cheese, ranch dressing, hot sauce and egg.
4. Mix well until combined and make 10 even sized meatballs. Place on baking tray.
5. Bake in preheated oven for 15 minutes.
6. Garnish with parsley and serve with sauce.

Nutritional Value (Amount per Serving):
- Calories 334
- Fat 14.1 g
- Carbohydrates 1.9 g
- Sugar 1.2 g
- Protein 47.1 g
- Cholesterol 200 mg

17-Quick and Tasty Chicken Salad

Total Time: 10 minutes

Serves: 4 Servings

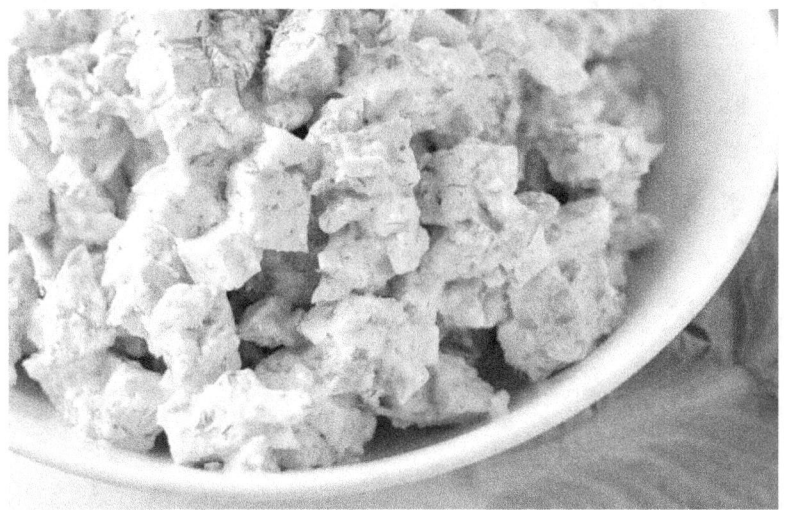

Ingredients:
- 1/2 lb chicken breast, cooked and cut into pieces
- 1 1/2 tablespoon fresh dill
- 1/2 tablespoon Dijon mustard
- 6 tablespoon mayonnaise
- 1 medium onion, chopped
- 4 tablespoon celery, diced
- Pepper
- Salt

Directions:

1. In mixing bowl, add all ingredients and mix well until combined.
2. Serve immediately and enjoy.

Nutritional Value (Amount per Serving):
- Calories 123
- Fat 8.4 g
- Carbohydrates 8.2 g
- Sugar 2.7 g
- Protein 4.0 g
- Cholesterol 15 mg

18-Delicious Chicken Broccoli Stir Fry

Total Time: 20 minutes

Serves: 4 Servings

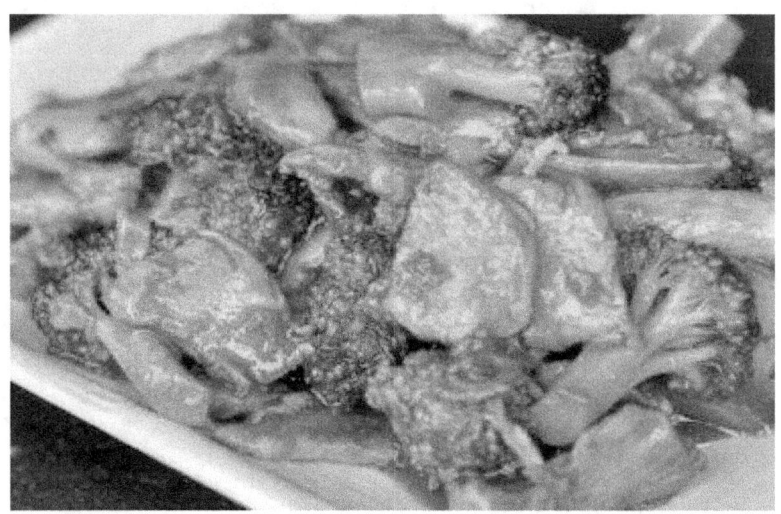

Ingredients:
- 1 lb chicken breast, skinless and boneless, cut into pieces
- 2 tsp cornstarch
- 2 cups broccoli florets
- 2 tsp sugar
- 2 tablespoon soy sauce
- 1 cup chicken stock
- 1 tsp ginger, chopped
- 3 garlic cloves, minced
- 1 tablespoon olive oil

Directions:

1. Heat olive oil in a pan over medium-high heat.
2. Add garlic, ginger and chicken and fry for 3 minutes or until chicken brown.
3. Add 3/4 cup chicken stock, sugar and soy sauce. Cover pan with lid and cook for 5 minutes. Stir well.
4. Add broccoli stir well. Cover and cook for 5 minutes or until broccoli tender.
5. Combine remaining chicken stock and cornstarch, stir into chicken broccoli mixture and cook until sauce thickens.
6. Serve hot and enjoy.

Nutritional Value (Amount per Serving):

- Calories 111
- Fat 5.5 g
- Carbohydrates 8.0 g
- Sugar 3.1 g
- Protein 8.4 g
- Cholesterol 19 mg

19-Spicy Grilled Chicken

Total Time: 25 minutes

Serves: 4 Servings

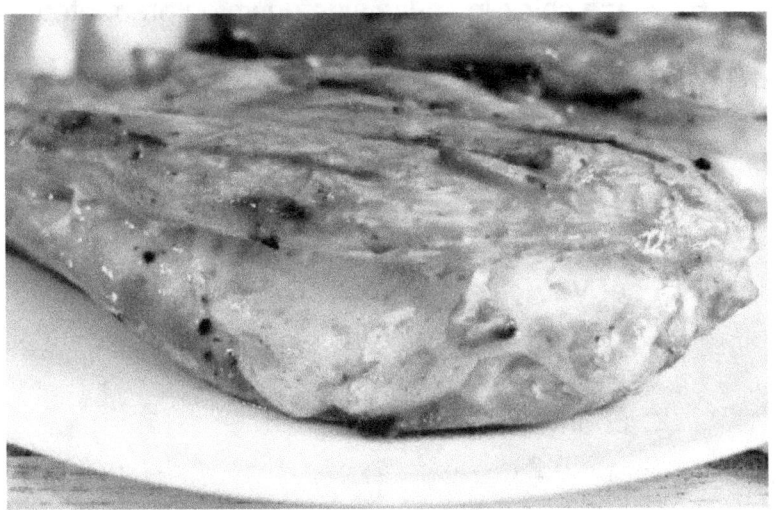

Ingredients:
- 1 lb chicken breast, boneless
- 4 tablespoon franks hot sauce
- 1 tsp butter, melted
- 4 tablespoon mozzarella cheese, shredded
- Pepper
- Salt

Directions:
1. Preheat the grill to medium heat.
2. Cut chickens horizontally, do not cut all the way.

3. Sprinkle black pepper inside the chicken then evenly top with shredded cheese.
4. In a small bowl, combine hot sauce, butter, and salt.
5. Spread the hot sauce and butter mixture on one side of chicken.
6. Place chicken sauce side down on preheated grill.
7. Then spread hot sauce and butter mixture over the top side of chicken cook for 7 minutes.
8. Turn chicken and cook for another 5 minutes.
9. Serve hot and enjoy.

Nutritional Value (Amount per Serving):
- Calories 130
- Fat 7.6 g
- Carbohydrates 1.0 g
- Sugar 0.2 g
- Protein 14.3 g
- Cholesterol 36 mg

20-Easy Slow Cooker Chicken Soup

Total Time: 3 hours 10 minutes

Serves: 4 Servings

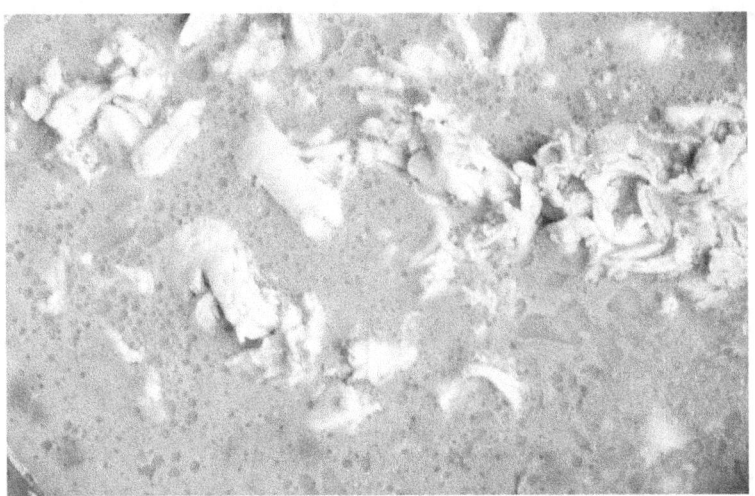

Ingredients:
- 1 lb chicken, boneless and skinless
- 6 oz pepper jack cheese, shredded
- 12 oz chicken stock
- 12 oz chunky salsa

Directions:
1. Add all ingredients into the slow cooker and mix well.
2. Cook on high for 3 hours.
3. Remove chicken and shred using a fork. Return shredded chicken into the slow cooker.
4. Serve hot and enjoy.

Nutritional Value (Amount per Serving):
- Calories 365
- Fat 17.4 g
- Carbohydrates 5.6 g
- Sugar 2.9 g
- Protein 45.0 g
- Cholesterol 133 mg

21-Yummy Sweet and Sour Chicken

Total Time: 55 minutes

Serves: 5 Servings

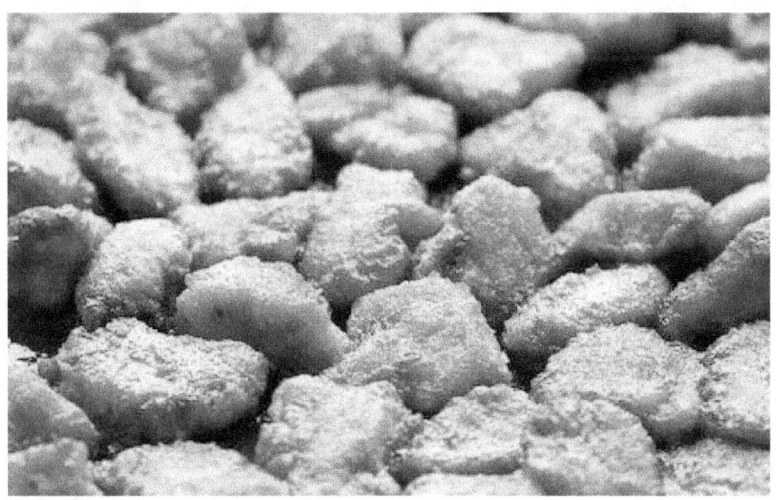

Ingredients:
- 3 lbs chicken wings, separate wings from drumette
- 4 chilies, chopped
- 4 tablespoon scallions, chopped
- 3 tablespoon granulated sugar substitute
- 1/4 cup water
- 2 tablespoon soy sauce
- 2 tsp vinegar
- 3 tablespoon rice vinegar
- 1/2 tsp sesame oil

Directions:

1. Place chicken wings on baking tray and bake at 375 F for 45 minutes.
2. Combine all remaining ingredients except scallions into the saucepan and bring to boil.
3. Simmer for 2 minutes until thickened. Remove pan from heat.
4. Once wings are cooked then add sauce mix well and boil for 2 minutes.
5. Garnish with scallions.
6. Serve hot and enjoy.

Nutritional Value (Amount per Serving):

- Calories 532
- Fat 20.6 g
- Carbohydrates 0.9 g
- Sugar 0.2 g
- Protein 79.2 g
- Cholesterol 240 mg

Chapter fourth beef Recipes

22-Low Carb Meatloaf

Total Time: 1 hour 10 minutes

Serves: 8 Servings

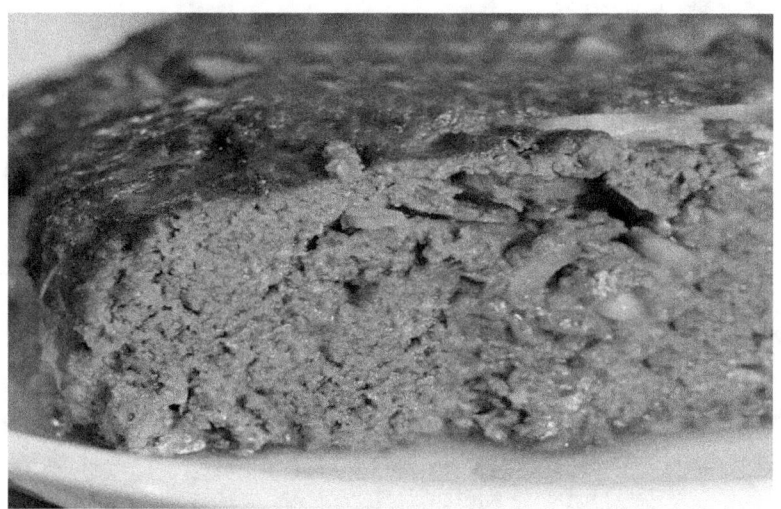

Ingredients:
- 2 large eggs
- 2 lbs ground beef
- 1 tsp garlic powder
- 1 small onion, chopped
- 1/2 cup parmesan cheese, grated
- 2 tsp salt

Directions:

1. In a mixing bowl, add all ingredients and mix well until combined.
2. Spray a loaf pan with cooking spray.
3. Add beef mixture into the loaf pan and bake at 350 F for 60 minutes.
4. Allow to cool for 10 minutes before slicing.
5. Serve with sauce and enjoy.

Nutritional Value (Amount per Serving):

- Calories 233
- Fat 8.3 g
- Carbohydrates 1.2 g
- Sugar 0.6 g
- Protein 36.1 g
- Cholesterol 148 mg

23-Spicy Stuffed Peppers

Total Time: 20 minutes

Serves: 6 Servings

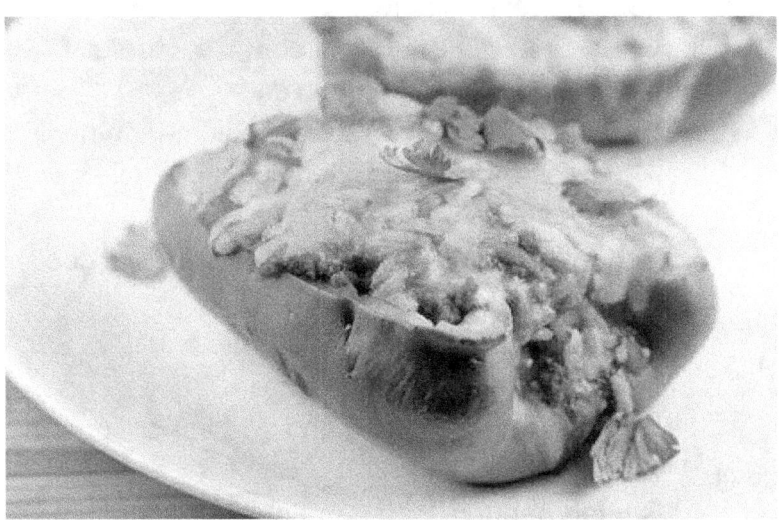

Ingredients:
- 1 lb ground beef
- 3 large green bell peppers, cut into the half
- 4 oz cheddar cheese, shredded
- 1/2 cup tomato puree
- 1/2 ground chipotle chili
- 1 tablespoon chili powder
- 1 tablespoon ground cumin
- 1 cup mushrooms, chopped
- 1 medium onion, chopped
- 2 tsp extra virgin olive oil

- 1/2 tsp salt

Directions:
1. Add 1 cup water in microwave-safe dish and place prepare bell peppers in dish.
2. Cover dish with plastic wrap and microwave peppers for 4 minutes.
3. Open plastic wrap and drain water carefully.
4. Flip peppers cut side up in dish.
5. Heat olive oil in a pan over medium-high heat.
6. Add beef and cook for 5 minutes or until browned.
7. Add mushrooms and onion. Stir well and cook for 5 minutes.
8. Add chipotle, chili powder, cumin and salt. Stir well and cook for 1 minute.
9. Remove pan from heat and add tomato puree. Mix well.
10. Stuffed peppers with meat mixture and top with shredded cheese.
11. Microwave the stuffed peppers for 2 minutes or until cheese melted.
12. Serve warm and enjoy.

Nutritional Value (Amount per Serving):
- Calories 274
- Fat 13.2 g
- Carbohydrates 9.8 g
- Sugar 5.2 g
- Protein 29.5 g
- Cholesterol 87 mg

24-Low Carb Beef Chili

Total Time: 6 hours 10 minutes

Serves: 6 Servings

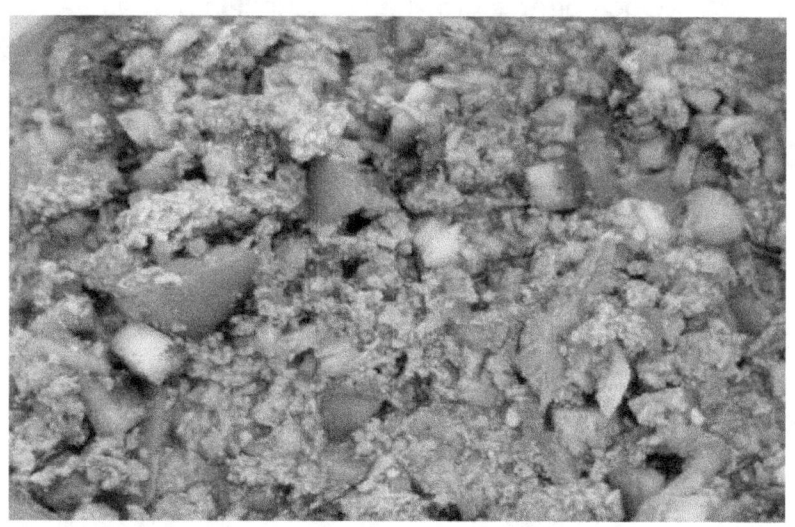

Ingredients:
- 1 lb ground beef
- 1 tsp garlic powder
- 1 tsp paprika
- 3 tsp chili powder
- 1 tablespoon Worcestershire sauce
- 1 tablespoon parsley, chopped
- 1 tsp onion powder
- 24 oz tomatoes, chopped
- 4 carrots, chopped
- 1 large onion, chopped

- 1 bell pepper, seeded and chopped
- 1/2 tsp salt

Directions:
1. Add ground beef in pan and brown over high heat.
2. Once beef is browned, spoon it into slow cooker.
3. Now add all remaining ingredients into the slow cooker and mix well until combined.
4. Cover slow cooker with lid and cook on high for 6 hours.
5. Stir well and serve hot.

Nutritional Value (Amount per Serving):
- Calories 205
- Fat 5.3 g
- Carbohydrates 14.4 g
- Sugar 7.9 g
- Protein 25.1 g
- Cholesterol 68 mg

25-Healthy Beef and Broccoli Stir Fry

Total Time: 20 minutes

Serves: 4 Servings

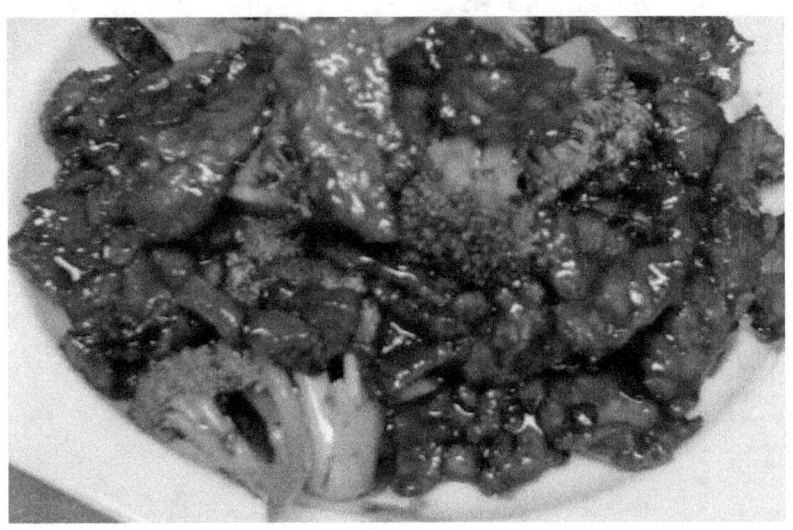

Ingredients:
- 1 lb lean beef, cut into slices
- 3 cups broccoli florets
- 3 scallions, chopped
- 1/2 cup parsley, chopped
- 2 red peppers, sliced
- 1 tsp ginger
- 1 tsp Dijon mustard
- 1 tsp garlic, minced
- 1 tsp sesame oil
- 2 tablespoon water

- 2 tablespoon soy sauce
- 1 tsp olive oil

Directions:
1. In mixing bowl, add beef slices, mustard, ginger, garlic, oil, water, and soy sauce. Mix well and set aside.
2. Heat olive oil in a pan over high heat.
3. Add pepper and broccoli and cook until tender and crisp.
4. Add beef slice mixture and cook until doneness.
5. Add parsley and scallions. Stir well.
6. Serve and enjoy.

Nutritional Value (Amount per Serving):
- Calories 277
- Fat 9.9 g
- Carbohydrates 9.0 g
- Sugar 2.8 g
- Protein 37.8 g
- Cholesterol 101 mg

26-Tasty Beef Roast

Total Time: 6 hours 10 minutes

Serves: 4 Servings

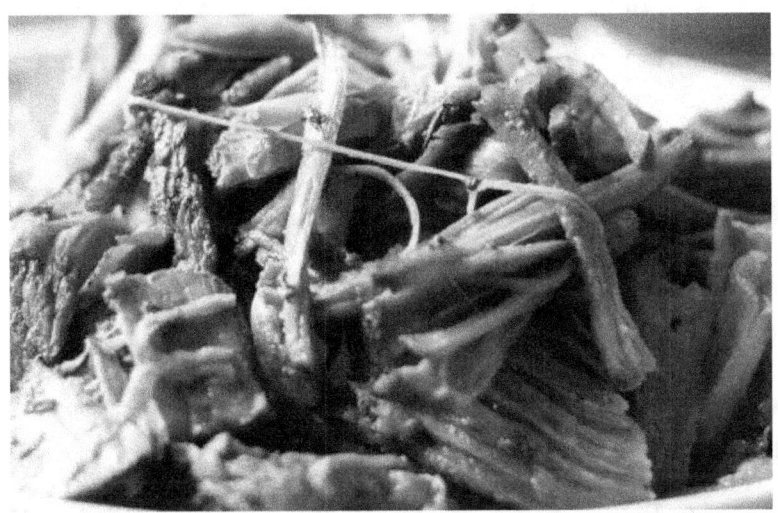

Ingredients:
- 1 1/4 lbs beef round roast
- 1/4 tsp marjoram
- 1/4 tsp thyme
- 1/2 tsp basil
- 4 tablespoon red wine
- 1/4 cup water
- 1 small onion, sliced
- 1/4 tsp black pepper
- 1/2 tsp salt

Directions:

1. In a small bowl, combine all spices and set aside.
2. Place beef roast in the bottom of slow cooker.
3. Sprinkle spice mixture over the beef roast. Add onion, water, and red wine.
4. Cook on low for 6 hours or until meat starts falling apart.
5. Once meat is cooked, shred with fork and mix with juices.
6. Serve and enjoy.

Nutritional Value (Amount per Serving):
- Calories 283
- Fat 8.8 g
- Carbohydrates 2.2 g
- Sugar 0.9 g
- Protein 43.2 g
- Cholesterol 127 mg

27-Low Carb Sweet and Spicy Beef

Total Time: 15 minutes

Serves: 4 Servings

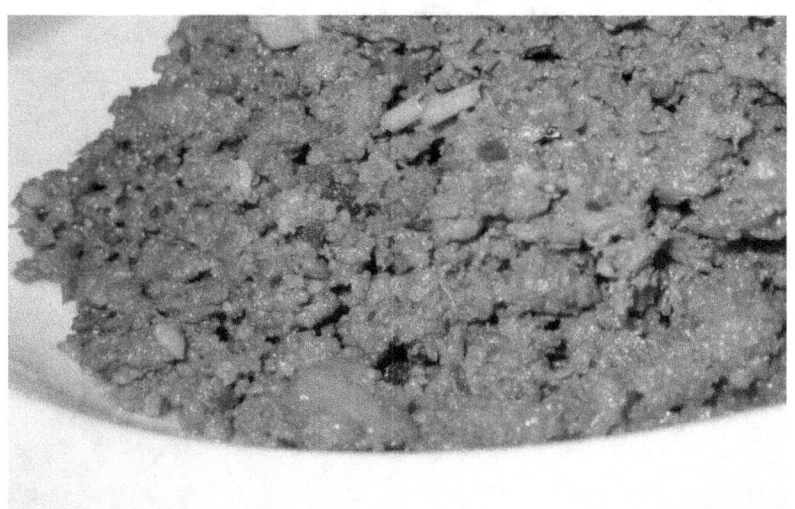

Ingredients:
- 1 lb ground beef
- 4 tablespoon green onion, sliced
- 1 tsp red pepper, crushed
- 1/2 tsp fresh ginger, minced
- 3 tablespoon soy sauce
- 1/2 tsp molasses
- 1/2 tsp stevia drops
- 2 garlic cloves, minced
- 1 tablespoon olive oil

Directions:

1. Heat olive oil in a pan over medium heat.
2. Once the oil is hot, add garlic and ground beef and cook until beef brown about 6 minutes.
3. Add red pepper, ginger, soy sauce, molasses, and stevia. Mix well.
4. Stir for 2 minutes until well blended.
5. Garnish with green onion and serve.

Nutritional Value (Amount per Serving):
- Calories 264
- Fat 10.7 g
- Carbohydrates 4.9 g
- Sugar 2.3 g
- Protein 35.7 g
- Cholesterol 101 mg

28-Delicious Sesame Beef Bowls

Total Time: 25 minutes

Serves: 4 Servings

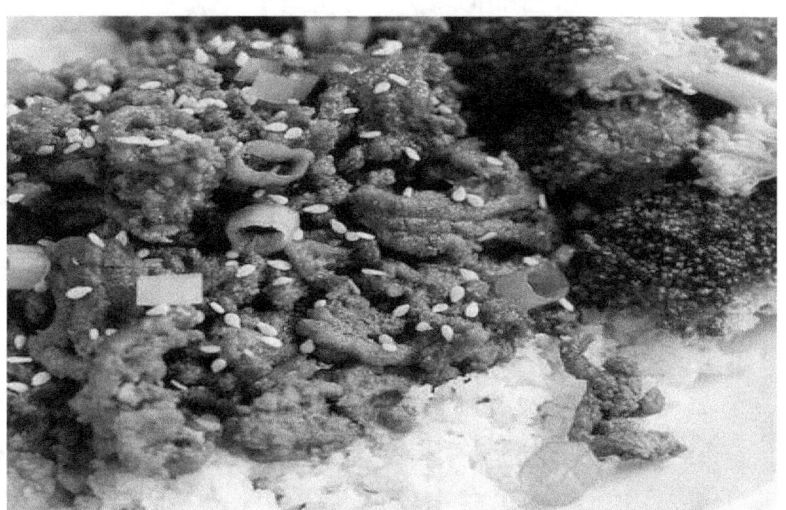

Ingredients:
- 1 1/2 lbs ground beef
- 1 lb broccoli florets, steamed
- 4 cups cauliflower rice
- 1 tablespoon sesame seeds, toasted
- 2 tablespoon olive oil
- 1/2 tsp chili paste
- 4 tablespoon scallions, chopped
- 1 tablespoon ginger, grated
- 3 garlic cloves, minced
- 2 tablespoon sesame oil
- 2 tablespoon honey

- 5 tablespoon coconut amino
- 1/2 tsp pepper

Directions:
1. In a small bowl, combine chili paste, pepper, scallion, ginger, sesame oil, honey and coconut amino.
2. Heat olive oil in a pan over medium-high heat.
3. Add beef and cook for 8 minutes or until cook.
4. Add chili paste mixture and mix well until combined. Cover pan with lid and simmer for 4 minutes.
5. Serve with steamed broccoli and cauliflower rice.

Nutritional Value (Amount per Serving):
- Calories 532
- Fat 26.1 g
- Carbohydrates 19.3 g
- Sugar 10.9 g
- Protein 55.6 g
- Cholesterol 152 mg

Chapter five Lamb Recipes

29-Slow Cooker Lamb Roast

Total Time: 4 hours 10 minutes

Serves: 6 Servings

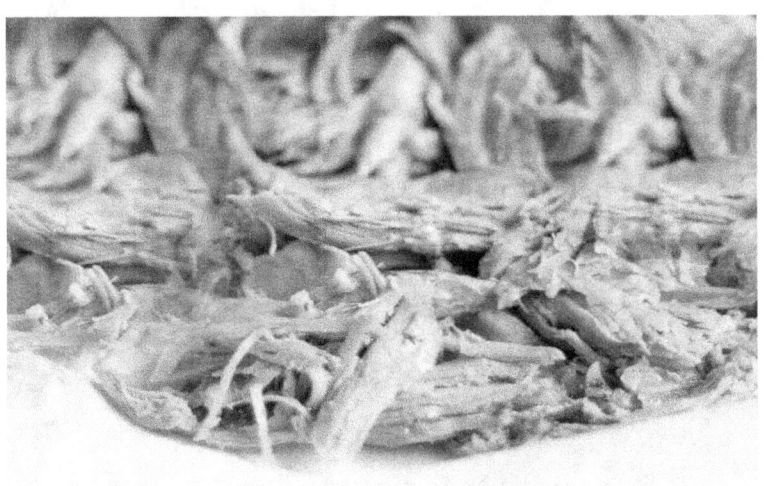

Ingredients:
- 4 lbs lamb leg
- 1 fresh lemon juice
- 1 tablespoon olive oil
- 4 tablespoon rosemary
- 4 garlic cloves, sliced
- Pepper
- Salt

Directions:

1. Make a deep incision all over the lamb legs.
2. Push rosemary and garlic into the incisions.
3. Pour olive oil over the lamb leg.
4. Season with pepper and salt.
5. Place seasoned lamb leg in a slow cooker.
6. Pour lemon juice over the lamb leg.
7. Cook lamb on high for 4 hours or until lamb easily shredded.
8. Serve and enjoy.

Nutritional Value (Amount per Serving):
- Calories 593
- Fat 24.8 g
- Carbohydrates 2.1 g
- Sugar 0.2 g
- Protein 85.1 g
- Cholesterol 272 mg

30-Low Carb Lamb Chops

Total Time: 25 minutes

Serves: 4 Servings

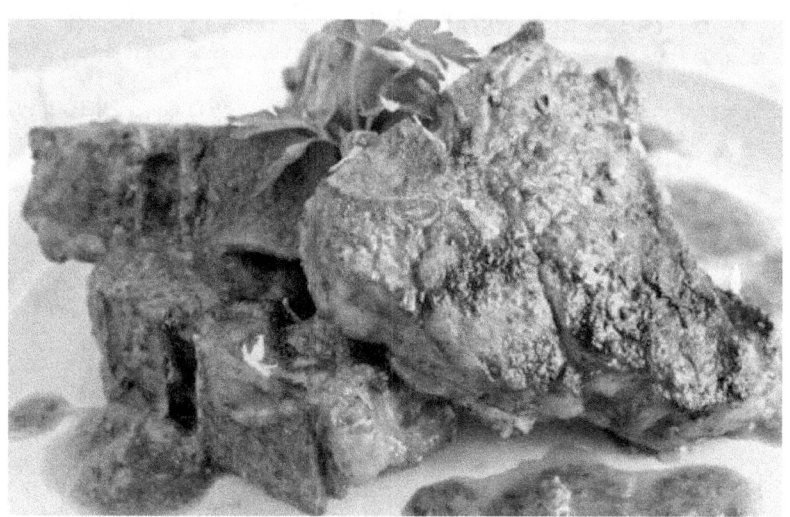

Ingredients:
- 1 rack of lamb
- 1 fresh lemon juice
- 1/2 cup olive oil
- 1/2 cup pine nuts
- 4 cups basil leaves
- 2 tablespoon ghee
- Pepper
- Salt

Directions:
1. Preheat the oven to 350 F.

2. Melt ghee in an oven safe pan over medium-high heat.
3. Season lamb with pepper and salt.
4. Once ghee is melted, add lamb and sear it for one minute.
5. Rotate lamb and seared from all sides.
6. Place pan with lamb in preheated oven and bake for 10 minutes.
7. Once it is done, remove from oven and place on cutting board. Allow to cool for few minutes.
8. Add lemon juice, olive oil, pine nuts, basil, pepper and salt in blender, and blend until smooth.
9. Now slice lamb and top with pesto.
10. Serve immediately and enjoy.

Nutritional Value (Amount per Serving):
- Calories 603
- Fat 51.6 g
- Carbohydrates 2.9 g
- Sugar 0.7 g
- Protein 35.0 g
- Cholesterol 118 mg

31-Spicy Pan Seared Lamb Chops

Total Time: 30 minutes

Serves: 5 Servings

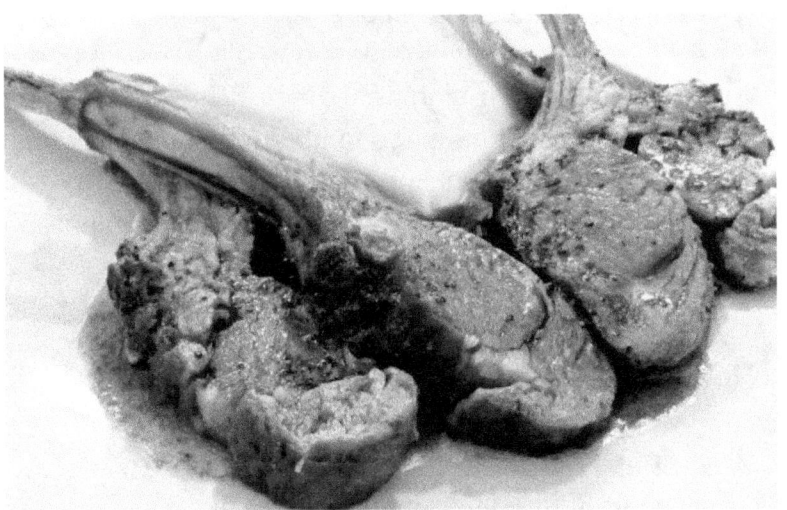

Ingredients:

- 5 lamb rib chops
- 2 tablespoon olive oil
- 1 tsp hot paprika
- 1/2 tsp smoked paprika
- 1 tsp cumin
- 1/2 tablespoon oregano
- 1 garlic clove, grated

Directions:

1. In a small bowl, combine hot paprika, smoked paprika, cumin, oregano, garlic and 1 tablespoon olive oil.
2. In mixing bowl, add lamb chops and paprika mixture rub until well coated and place in refrigerator for 3 hours.
3. Preheat the oven to 352 F.
4. Heat remaining 1 tablespoon olive oil in a pan over medium-high heat.
5. Once oil is hot, place lamb chops and cook for 3 minutes or until browned.
6. Flip chops to other side and bake in preheated oven for 8 minutes.
7. Serve hot and enjoy.

Nutritional Value (Amount per Serving):
- Calories 221
- Fat 12.4 g
- Carbohydrates 0.8 g
- Sugar 0.2 g
- Protein 25.7 g
- Cholesterol 82 mg

32-Low Carb Grilled Lamb Chops

Total Time: 25 minutes

Serves: 6 Servings

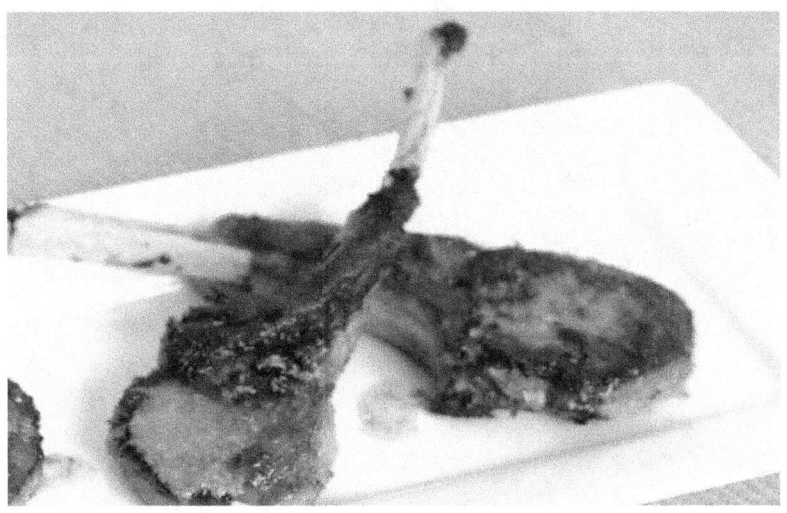

Ingredients:
- 6 lamb chops
- 1 tablespoon parsley, chopped
- 2 garlic cloves, minced
- 2 tablespoon ginger, minced
- 4 tablespoon olive oil
- 2 tablespoon coconut amino
- Pepper
- Salt

Directions:
1. Preheat the grill to medium-high heat.

2. In a bowl, combine parsley, garlic, ginger, olive oil, and coconut amino.
3. Add lamb chops in a bowl and mix until well coated.
4. Season lamb chops with pepper and salt.
5. Place lamb chops on preheated grill and grill for 4 minutes per side.
6. Allow to cool for 5 minutes then serve.

Nutritional Value (Amount per Serving):
- Calories 229
- Fat 15.0 g
- Carbohydrates 1.7 g
- Sugar 0.2 g
- Protein 21.5 g
- Cholesterol 68 mg

33-Simple Pan Seared Lamb Steaks

Total Time: 25 minutes

Serves: 4 Servings

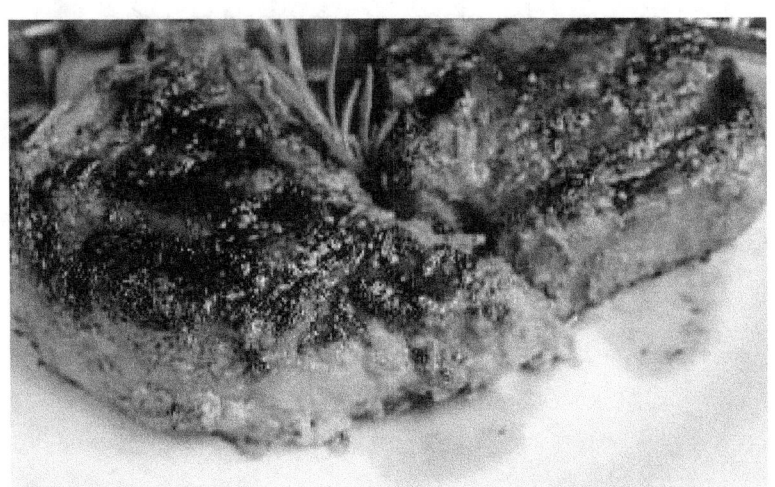

Ingredients:
- 4 lamb steaks
- 1 tablespoon olive oil
- 4 tsp thyme, minced
- 1 tsp onion powder
- 1 tsp garlic powder
- 1 tsp pepper
- 1 tsp kosher salt

Directions:
1. Season lamb with onion powder, garlic powder, pepper, and salt.
2. Heat olive oil in a pan over medium-high heat.

3. Once oil is hot, place season lamb steaks and cook for 2 minutes or until browned.
4. Turn to other side and cook for another 2 minutes.
5. Reduce heat to medium and again flip steaks and cook for 5 minutes.
6. Turn steaks once and cook for 4 minutes.
7. Garnish with thyme and serve.

Nutritional Value (Amount per Serving):
- Calories 249
- Fat 11.9 g
- Carbohydrates 2.0 g
- Sugar 0.2 g
- Protein 32.2 g
- Cholesterol 102 mg

34-Easy Low Carb Lamb Patties

Total Time: 30 minutes

Serves: 5 Servings

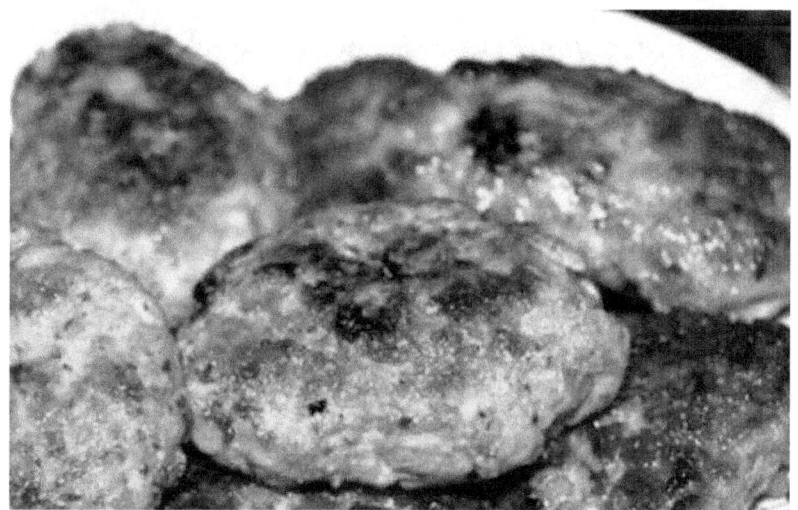

Ingredients:
- 1 lb ground lamb
- 1 large egg
- 1/2 tsp rosemary, chopped
- 1/2 tablespoon parsley, chopped
- 1 tsp ground cumin
- 5 oz halloumi cheese, grated
- 1/2 tsp pepper
- 1/4 tsp salt

Directions:

1. In mixing bowl, add all ingredients and mix until combined.
2. Make five even sized round shape patties from mixture.
3. Grill patties over medium-high heat for 5 minutes on each side.
4. Serve hot and enjoy.

Nutritional Value (Amount per Serving):
- Calories 289
- Fat 16.2 g
- Carbohydrates 1.2 g
- Sugar 0.8 g
- Protein 33.0 g
- Cholesterol 141 mg

35-Delicious Grilled Lamb Kebabs

Total Time: 30 minutes

Serves: 4 Servings

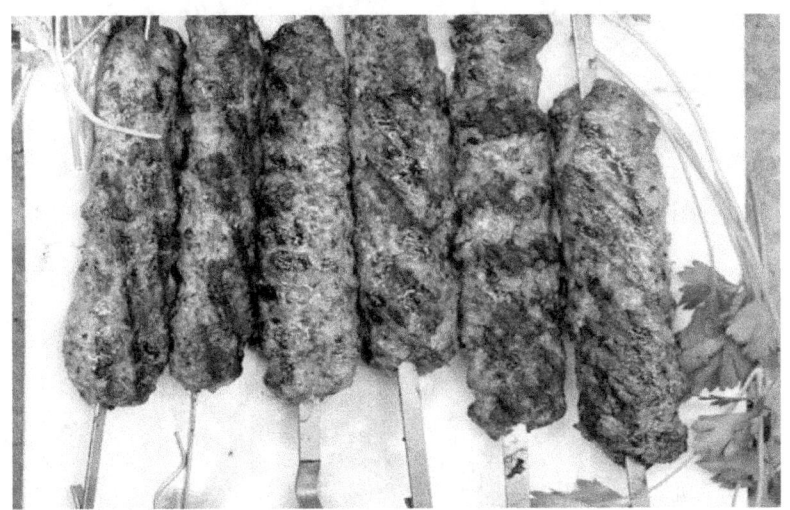

Ingredients:
- 1 lb ground lamb
- 1/4 tsp all spice mix
- 1/4 tsp ground cinnamon
- 4 tablespoon parsley, chopped
- 1 garlic clove, minced
- 1 medium onion, minced
- 1/4 tsp pepper
- 1/2 tsp salt

Directions:
1. Preheat the grill to medium-high heat.

2. In large mixing bowl, add all ingredients and mix until well combined.
3. Divide lamb mixture evenly in four portions and shape each portion into a sausage shape.
4. Thread lamb mixture onto a metal skewer.
5. Oil grills rack.
6. Place lamb skewer on hot grill and turn every 3 minutes until cooked about 10 minutes.
7. Allow to cool for 5 minutes then slice and serve.

Nutritional Value (Amount per Serving):
- Calories 225
- Fat 8.4 g
- Carbohydrates 3.2 g
- Sugar 1.2 g
- Protein 32.3 g
- Cholesterol 102 mg

for any reparation, damages, or monetary loss due to the information herein, either directly or indirectly. Respective authors own all copyrights not held by the publisher.

The information herein is offered for informational purposes solely and is universal as so. The presentation of the information is without contract or any type of guarantee assurance.

The trademarks that are used are without any consent, and the publication of the trademark is without permission or backing by the trademark owner. All trademarks and brands within this book are for clarifying purposes only and are the owned by the owners themselves, not affiliated with this document.

www.ingramcontent.com/pod-product-compliance
Lightning Source LLC
Chambersburg PA
CBHW060205290526
45789CB00003B/1173